WEIGHT LOSS – IT'S JUST NUTS!!

A Simple Plan You Can Do

By

Bob Binder

Acknowledgments

I would like to thank Lucile Puett for her patience, support, and input on this book, which helped to get it done, and it wouldn't be done without Lucy's help.

DEDICATION

This book is dedicated to my two adult daughters, Margaux Binder and Paige Binder.

WEIGHT LOSS – IT'S JUST NUTS!!
A Simple Plan You Can Do

Overview

You have just started on your own weight loss program by reading this and following these simple and easy ways to shed the extra pounds. This is about a relationship with yourself.

I lost 35 pounds, going from 197 to 162 pounds using this plan, and have kept off the weight that I lost, staying within a 5 pound range of 160 to 165 pounds. You can, too. And I don't intend to add it back on. That's over 17% of my weight. You can do that, or more.

This plan will guide you to take off your extra pounds and keep them off.

Other ways worked for me for awhile, but the pounds kept finding their way back. You probably have done so, too. Just follow these principles, and your weight will go down till you reach your goal and you can then keep it down as easily as possible.

This is not a quick weight loss plan. There are no tricks, no pills, no gum, no magic, no subscription sales, no surgery, no odd things to eat or drink. And the weight stays off, unlike the quick weight loss plans and the gimmick plans, which become quick gain-it-all-back plans.

Why is this book so short? So you can read the whole thing fairly quickly and get started right away. Keeping the plan simple makes it easier to follow and stay on.

There are 3 components to the *Weight Loss – It's Just Nuts* plan: fewer calories, eating healthier but good tasting foods you like, not bad tasting foods that you don't like, and more exercise, even if it's light exercise such as walking more.

Few people lose weight and keep it off by exercise alone or watching calories alone. This plan is a balanced combination of the two in a way that you can do and keep doing.

This is not a difficult program, and it's not easy or you would have done it already. But it can be done. All it takes is your willingness to do it. Nothing will do it for you – not pills, not machines, not your best friends or spouse, not complaining, not excuses. Just you.

After you get started and see this weight loss plan working, you'll get a new sense of personal accomplishment, a spring in your step, you'll walk straighter and taller, have better posture, feel better, have more energy, more self-esteem, better appearance – and a new sense of your own Will Power abilities.

This plan will work for you.

The amounts of calories are listed in some places. They are estimates, and they vary by size, portion, and other factors. Some of the sources disagreed on some of the calorie counts. The amounts stated are general estimates of what you can expect.

Online, the health benefits of some are for larger quantities. The quantities here are balanced, so you can get some of a lot of healthy things instead of a lot of one or two. And so the food portion is not huge.

Several products are mentioned by brand. None has paid a cent or offered anything in return for their mention. They are simply from my experience, and they are not meant to say that only that brand works. The brands are only to guide those who would like to know.

The specifics can be varied, but the principles need to remain for the plan to work.

What You Will Need

1.   A **scale.**

> Preferably a digital readout scale with 10ths of a pound. And it should measure body fat percentage. A good brand: Tanita (there are others)

> Weighing

> Weigh yourself at about the same time each day. The best time is after you get up in the morning, after any morning necessities, without clothes or watch, and before you have breakfast. That will be the most consistent and probably your lowest weight of the day. Keep track of it somewhere such as the following.

2.   An **app on your smart phone that keeps track of your weight**.

> Many good ones are free.

> Many will also keep track of your calories and exercise, so long as you enter them.

These apps will calculate how many calories you can have today based on your weight goal, today's weight, and exercise done, and it will vary some from day to day. These are guides more than precise numbers.

These apps will have calories for various foods, and you can add your own foods with calorie count, or summarize once you eat something regularly, such as any standard breakfasts you eat, if you have a similar combination of foods regularly. Pencil and paper will do, but an app on your smart phone will be more helpful.

You choose whether you want to lose ½ pound a week (that will take you a long time), a pound, 2 pounds, etc.

As you enter your food, drink, or exercise information, the app calculates how many calories you have left for that day. It couldn't be much simpler.

Losing more than 2 pounds a week is a lot and hard to stay with. 1 to 2 pounds per week is a good place to start. If you start with 2 pounds a week, and this just isn't happy for you, cut it back to 1 or 1 ½ pounds per week. This weight loss plan is easy to stay with and works. Tailor it so it works for you.

Lose It is an app that works well, showing a graph of your weight so you can see your weight drop. Many others will do so also. Choose one that suits you.

3. A **teaspoon measurer**.

Any grocery store or kitchen products store has them.

4. **Pedometer or smart phone app that counts steps**.

> There are many free apps that count steps. iPhones have a step counter in the Health app that comes with the phone. Pacer is a good free app. It counts steps, flights of stairs walked up, and translates that to calories lost, which you can enter into Lose It, where you're keeping your daily calories count – and exercise calories subtract from food and drink calories! There are many others.

5. An adult portion of **Will Power**.

> Not Olympic sized, just a normal adult portion. If you don't think you have it, look more carefully, it's there. Use it.

What is Nice to Have

6. **2 large size pill holders**.

> Not giant, but large. Very convenient. They are explained under Breakfast.

7. **Small food scale**.

> Not necessary, but helpful in how much to prepare at home. For example, 2 oz. of dry pasta is 1 serving, about 200 calories.

What You Should Have Anyway

8.   Comfortable walking shoes.

They don't have to be exercise shoes, just shoes that are comfortable to walk in.

Chapter 1

What to Expect

There are several plans to lose weight quickly and many fad diets. This plan is not one of them.

Many are simply unhealthy, and most are temporary weight loss plans. This is a healthy weight loss plan that lasts and that you can live with indefinitely.

In a few days, your scale will tell you this is working.

Awhile longer, your clothes will tell you, as your belt needs a little more tightening than it did before, and your clothes fit more nicely on you. You'll start feeling good about yourself and your appearance. You'll have more energy.

A little later, your friends will start telling you you've lost weight.

So will your mirror.

And your inner you will be very happy with your body, your appearance, how you feel, and yourself for having done this task that few accomplish for very long.

Here's what we're going to do:

1. Have a good, healthy, tasty, filling, breakfast
2. Watch how much we eat (smaller portions) the rest of the day
3. Pay attention to what we eat and drink, both quantity and health benefit (or lack thereof).

4. Walk or other exercise a little more.
5. Lose weight steadily, look better, feel better, be healthier.

Here's what we're *not* going to do.

1. Lose weight rapidly. You'll lose weight from ½ pound to 2 pounds a week, depending on you and your choices. You didn't put it on overnight, you can't lose it overnight.
2. Engage in a fad diet
3. Go hungry.
4. Deprive yourself of the foods you want.

Remember this: Your body knows
every calorie you put into it,
every calorie you save, and
every calorie you burn in exercise.

You can't fool your body.

Chapter 2

Weight, Body Fat Percentage, and Body Mass Index (BMI)

First, you need to pick a target weight for you.

There are many charts of ideal weights, and unfortunately they vary too much from each other for me to recommend one. Some are lower than others and seem to me to be too low. Very few seem to be too high. Look around on the internet until you find one that seems right to you. That's not necessarily the one that indicates the highest ideal weight for you. Similarly, don't punish yourself by picking one that's unreasonably low.

Not too long from now, you'll reach the weight where you feel good, balanced, and that it's the right one for you. In the meantime, pick a realistic target weight, something you can do. You can revise it as you go or set a new one and lower it when you reach your initial target.

You can search online for "weight range chart" then click on images, and you will see a large number of charts. Click on these until you find one that makes sense for you.

The body fat percentage on your home scale will come with a chart. It is different for men and women, and you should consult that chart. It is similar to the BMI chart below but may or may not be exactly the same depending on gender, age, etc.

Body Mass Index is a measure of body fatness. The standard weight status categories associated with BMI ranges for adults are shown in the following table (Centers for Disease Control –

www.cdc.gov). There are many BMI calculators online to figure your BMI. You don't need to know the formula. You just put in your height and weight.

BMI	**Weight Status**
Below 18.5	Underweight
18.5 – 24.9	Normal or Healthy Weight
25.0 – 29.9	Overweight
30.00 and Above	Obese

Chapter 3

Weekday Breakfast

Let's get started.

<u>Breakfast</u>

This is the most important meal. This is a healthy, tasty, filling start to the day, and sets the stage for the rest of the day.

This is a breakfast you can eat 5 times or more a week and be happy with it.

Take a regular bowl for cereal (yes, cereal, but read this and taste it – you'll like it).

Have 4 kinds of cereal plus oatmeal (also a cereal) in your cupboard, all with whole grains as the main ingredient. All with 3 grams or more of fiber and 14 grams or less of sugar and 180 calories or less per cup.

Have one basic, fairly low calorie cereal, such as Cheerios (original) in your cupboard.

Now here's a good, healthy, filling, tasty breakfast, a total of about 485 healthy, filling, tasty calories. You may like it as is or adapt it for your own tastes.

The Cereals:

All are whole grain. All General Mills cereals are whole grain. Other brands have whole grain cereals as well.

All have information regarding calories, fiber, and sugar on the box, sometimes on the front. Look at the ingredients chart on the cereal box in the store. The first ingredient should be a whole grain. Whole grain wheat and oats are good choices.

Or, you can substitute Oatmeal such as Quaker Maple Brown Sugar Instant Lower Sugar Oatmeal (120 calories, 3 g fiber, 4 g sugar).

1/4 cup Cheerios (or other basic cereal), 1/4 cup one of the others (for health and taste)

Calories – about 140 Calories, Fiber, Sugar

Cheerios (original)	110 calories/cup, 3 g fiber, 1.2 g sugar
Fiber One Honey Clusters	170 calories/cup, 10 g fiber, 9 g sugar
Fiber One Raisin Bran Clusters	170 calories/cup, 10 g fiber, 14 g sugar
Trader Joe's High Fiber Fruit & Nut Multigrain Medley	135 calories/cup, 7 g fiber, 8 g sugar

The Raw Nuts (Unsalted, Unroasted):

You can get these in any quantity you want in bulk at Whole Foods, some health food stores, HEB and Central Market stores in Texas. Many other groceries have bulk food areas now.

Calories – about 89

1 Cashew	9
1 Pecan half	10
1 Walnut half	13
1 small Macadamia or ½ large one	19
1 Almond (blanched or not)	7
1 Brazil Nut half	15
5 Pistachios (shelled is easier)	16

The Raw Seeds (Unsalted, Unroasted) plus Oat Bran and Cranberries:

1 *level* teaspoon each. Not a heaping teaspoon, a level one.

Calories – about 89

Oat Bran	12
Sunflower	17
Pumpkin	15
Flax	15
Chia	22
Dried Cranberries	8

The Fruit (One of These at Breakfast):

You can add ½ banana sliced in your cereal or on the side – very tasty – and put the other ½ banana (not yet sliced) in a baggie in the refrigerator for the next day. The other fruits are delicious as well, adding taste and health benefits, apple and pear go great in or out of the cereal. If you make pancakes, banana, apple, blueberries, seeds, or nuts go well in pancakes.

<u>Calories – about 50</u>

½ Banana (Medium or Large)	50
½ Apple	58
½ Pear	50
1 cup Watermelon, diced	46
½ Grapefruit (Large)	52

Other, in Cereal:

<u>Calories – about 54</u>

½ cup Skim Milk	45
Blueberries (10-12)	9

Other, Not in Cereal:

<u>Calories – about 63</u>

Prune	20
3 Grapes	9
1 capsule Fish Oil (Nordic Naturals Ultimate Omega + CoQ10)	10
Dark Chocolate (small piece, Size of dime to quarter) (Trader Joe's Swiss 72%)	24

The Combination:

Calories – about 485 total

If you have sweetened coffee or juice for breakfast, you will need to add those calories in as well. Everything counts.

Later, After Your Weight is Under Control:

After breakfast, a little bite of something sweet (Optional, when your weight loss has started and is under control):

Don't start adding these till you have a substantial and regular weight loss or you've reached a maintenance state. These will bring your breakfast calorie count to about 530 calories.

Calories – about 45

Cookie (small bite)	25
2 or 3 Trader Joe's Sesame Honey Cashews	20

Now you have a variable, delicious, healthy breakfast. Yes, healthy. Yes, delicious. Yes, variable, not the same every day. As you can see you can tailor this to what you like, deleting a few things, adding a few things. There are many different and good flavors and textures, and everything is a healthy bite, tastes great, and is good for you.

Putting It All Together:

Here's how you put it all together:

1. Put 1/4 cup of Cheerios and 1/4 cup of any of the other 3 cereals into the bowl
    > (1/4 cup is about a small handful, not a medium or large handful, a small handful – measure with a measuring cup the first time, and see what it feels and looks like)
    Or pre-measured bag of instant Oatmeal
2. Add Nuts
3. Add Seeds plus Oat Bran and Dried Cranberries
4. Add Blueberries
5. Add Banana slices or Pear chunks or Apple chunks to the cereal.
    Or Watermelon or Grapefruit on the side.
6. Add Milk
7. On the side: Grapes, Prune, Fish Oil, Dark Chocolate

To Make Adding the Nuts, Seeds, Oat Bran, and Cranberries Easier:

This is where the 2 large 7-day pill holders come in.

Once a week, pre-pack in each of the 7 daily compartments the daily amount of nuts in one pill holder and the seeds plus oat bran and dried cranberries in the other, and you have a very quick way to add the nuts and seeds and dried cranberries in the morning. Plus, they are easy to carry with you on trips.

Grabbing Breakfast on the Run:

Sometimes, you have to grab a quick breakfast in a fast food place. Take your nuts, seeds, and dried cranberries in a baggie (easy to do from the weekly pill holders you have them in). In another baggie, take your prune, dark chocolate, fish oil capsule, and grapes. Take ½ a banana.

The ½ banana you can eat in the car, on the train, bus, beside the breakfast, or whatever. Also, the banana will pick up your seeds, oat bran, and dried cranberries if you want to press them together and eat them that way. Just dip the banana into a pile of them or into the baggie.

The rest, you take in to the breakfast place. Simply add the first baggie to your oatmeal or cereal, or put on the side of your plate. If on the side, you can easily put the seeds, oat bran, and dried cranberries on a lightly buttered or jellied piece of (hopefully whole wheat) toast and eat the nuts with your fingers. The other baggie, put the contents on your plate or napkin and eat as usual.

Chapter 4

Lunch

This is a hard one to keep under control, as most people don't have a lot of choices for lunch and restaurants serve too much. Try to stay around 500 calories or less. Many more restaurants are listing calories on their menus. Also, many restaurants have their calories online -- just search the restaurant's name and the word "nutrition." You can also get a general idea of the calories in a type of meal by looking it up on your smart phone.

Don't order giant things. If you do, divide your food in half and take the other half home. Try to go to restaurants where the menu has the calories on it or where you know ahead of time the approximate calories.

The important thing is to downsize. If you end up at a hamburger place, tear off and throw away the unnecessary bun. The bun usually has little nutrition. Get a whole wheat bun, if offered.

If it's a big, calorie laden plate, simply don't eat all of it.

Remember this: You've already agreed to pay for the lunch.
You save no money by eating it all.
Nor do you feed any hungry people anywhere in the world by
*   eating it all.*
Eat only what is good for you and gets rid of that hungry
*   feeling.*

If it's a high calorie lunch, eat less than the whole meal – half the meal, or at most 2/3. How do you do this? You divide the meal into halves or 2/3 *as soon as you get it* and either take the rest home or throw it away. Again, you save not a cent by eating it all.

Once you've eaten that which you agreed with yourself to eat, put the rest in a take home container, throw it away, cover it up with the paper it came in, or move it far away from you. Don't nibble on it. Don't count on eating just half or 2/3 if you don't divide it up at first.

A few suggestions: Club sandwich (easy to take some home). Chicken and turkey sandwiches, with little mayonnaise (if too much, soak up excess with a napkin and throw it away). Panera Bread ½ sandwich. Subway (many good choices). McDonald's McChicken – 380 calories. Schlotzky's small, smoked turkey on whole wheat – 353 calories. Whataburger, Jr. – 310 calories. Many other choices.

French fries? These are your enemies. Little health benefit. Large calorie count. But they taste good, darn it. McDonald's small fries alone are 230 calories. If you must, limit yourself to 10 small thin fries, 5 of the larger cut fries.

Chips and salsa? Chips are about 10 calories each. Limit yourself to 5.

Chips and queso? Ha! Maybe 3 chips with a *little* queso on them, not a lot of queso, a little. This is very easy to overdo.

Chapter 5

Dinner (Supper in the parts of the South and Texas)

This should be eaten as early as you feel comfortable eating it, so that your body metabolism, your walking, moving around the house, walking the dog, or other exercise continues to burn up calories from dinner before bedtime. Eating just before bedtime puts you in bed with all that food ready to be made into fat.

You can make dinner at home. It's less expensive, usually healthier, and you can make what and how much you want.

Suggestions:

Bacon, Lettuce, and Tomato sandwich. Go easy on the mayonnaise. Add an avocado slice for taste or health. Whole wheat bread, of course.

Ham sandwich. Thin slice or slices (about 1or 2 oz.), plus lettuce and tomato.

Spaghetti or other Pasta. Noodles have about 200 calories (2 oz. dry). So, be careful on the sauce. Read the labels, and then make it taste better with what you like. Slice some more tomatoes in it, or mushrooms, or black olives, or red bell peppers, or onions, etc. You can really get creative easily here. Go easy on the Parmesan cheese. Make your own garlic bread. Go easy on the butter or margarine (a good one is Healthy Choice with Olive Oil), add Italian spices and granulated garlic or garlic powder.

Be creative. Have what you want, just learn to estimate what will be about 500 - 600 calories total.

You can even have a little dessert, if you can limit it to a few bites.

Chapter 6

Other Eating Out and Weekends

This is where you make up for depriving yourself, if you feel deprived. Go where you want, order what you want, within reason, and split it with you wife/husband/friend/significant other/or whoever will split it with you. Or, if no one, split it with yourself, take the rest home, and have it another day (this gives you 2 meals, so each meal costs you half as much).

Eggs are only 80 - 100 calories each and healthy. Bread has about 65 calories per slice before you put anything on it. So, a couple of eggs and toast with a little butter and jelly. Migas (skip the tortilla), Taco (whole wheat tortilla, if available). 2 pancakes instead of 3 (go easy on the butter and syrup). Oatmeal. Split an Eggs Benedict with someone.

A late breakfast-lunch combination is an excellent treat. If you can wait for breakfast till about 11 am, you can have more calories than either alone, as you're having both breakfast and lunch (but not as much as both together). This is a meal you can look forward to and have a lot of flexibility with.

Eating out is a time for something a little different, just don't overdo it.

A good thing to do is split meals with your significant other. Mine regularly splits meals with me, as many meals are just too darn big, and she noticed my weight loss! It helps. PS Don't forget to tip the waitperson as if you got two entrees, as he/she did the same work as serving you two entrees even though it was split.

Dinner is similar – don't overdo it. Keep in mind what you've already had today. If you had a light breakfast and lunch or light breakfast-lunch combination, you have more flexibility in what you can have for dinner.

Remember this: No cheating.
Any cheating is cheating yourself. No one else. Just you.

Chapter 7

Exercise

This is as much part of your weight loss program as watching calories. Exercise not only burns calories, but it keeps burning them for a good while after you are no longer exercising. In addition, over time, you will develop more muscles where you concentrate your exercise – and muscle tissue burns more calories than fat tissue.

Walking

Just walk more. Your body wants you to walk more, your significant other wants you to walk more, you want you to walk more, everyone wants you to walk more.

This is the easiest to add to your schedule and life.

Use your pedometer or smart phone step counter.

Most people walk about 3,000 steps a day. 10,000 steps a day is the ideal number. But for most people, that's unrealistic without devoting a lot of time to it. This is more easily achievable on vacation, particularly when out sightseeing or exploring a new place.

So, first find out how many steps a day you're taking for the first couple of days or so. Then bump that up by 500 or 1,000 steps per day for a week or two. Then, add another 500 or 1,000 steps per day. The realistic goal is to get at least 4,000 steps per day, 5,000 steps if you can, and hopefully 6,000 steps.

Most people walk about a mile in 2,000 to 2,400 steps, depending on their stride.

Walk the dog a little farther. Park across the lot at the grocery store, movie, shopping mall, work, Home Depot, wherever.   Walk to the mailbox instead of driving to it. Your body knows you've helped it.

Also, walk a little more briskly than usual. No strolling or meandering along, except in those special, beautiful times when you're enjoying your surroundings alone or with your special one.

Other Exercise

If walking is not something you want to do more of, or you simply want to vary the type of exercise your body gets (an excellent thing to do), find something that appeals to you. It doesn't have to be a lot. Anything helps.

Set aside actual walking or jogging time. 10 minutes a day is better than what you may be doing. 20 minutes is even better.   Your body knows everything you do. Get up out of your chair more often, even if just to get another glass of water.

Do sit-ups, crunches, push-ups, weights, squats, or whatever you're willing to do.

Lift 5, 10, 15, 20 pound weights, or whatever suits you, a large number of times.

You can walk, jog, dance, swim, bicycle, stretch, do yoga, work in the garden, lift a few weights, whatever you like. Just do something more than what you've been doing.

You can get in 15 or 20 minutes or more of exercise and stretching just before going to bed if you can't find another time – some of it while on the bed, such as stretching, light crunches, pulling knee up, etc. While it may be better to do all this on the floor, doing it on the bed is better than not doing it at all.

Going to another floor at work? Take the stairs, if it's not too many flights. Make 2 trips bringing the groceries in instead of carrying too much at once.   Just add things here and there. It all adds up.

The point is: Do Something More Than What You're Doing.

Beverage After Exercise

Don't forget to drink plenty of water when you exercise.

If you lose a lot of sweat through exercise or heat, a good replenishment drink such as Gatorade will help restore lost potassium and energy. It does have calories, keep in mind, except water, which has no calories and is very, very good for you.

Chapter 8

Water, Beverages, Salted Foods, Binging, Snacks, Candy Bars, etc.

Go easy on all of these, except water. Don't binge eat. You can undo a lot of good you have done with too much food or too much of the wrong kind of food.

Calories

Coca-Cola 12 oz	140 (that's a lot)
Coca-Cola McDonald's Medium	220 (that's a whole lot)
Beer (varies a good bit) 12 oz can	150 (that's where beer bellies can come from)
Light Beer 12 oz can (varies)	110
White Wine 5 oz (varies)	120
Red Wine 6 oz (served larger) varies	150

Water

Water is the premier health food. We're made of this. Drink a lot of water (not all at once, of course). Keep water near you at home, at work, in your car, and bedside, if you want.

There are many drinking containers that keep drinks cool (or warm) for long periods of time, and they're great for keeping ice water handy. These same containers will usually keep drinks warm, but for a somewhat shorter period of time.

Yeti brand 20 oz tumbler is very good, versatile, and easy to use. It really will keep ice all day in your beverage.

Salted Foods

I'm sure you noticed that all the seeds and nuts were raw. And you've noticed that the seeds and nuts in little packages are salted. Watch out for those. Salt makes you thirsty, you drink more Coke, beer, whatever, and you retain water. The water will go away in a day or two, but you're adding an unnecessary burden on your weight loss efforts with salt. If you do it every day, well, the extra weight just remains.

You will get plenty of salt in your everyday eating, many times what you need. Salt has other health hazards for some, but I'm sticking to the weight aspect.

Almost all snack foods, restaurant foods, canned foods, pizzas – you name it – have way more salt than you need (listed as sodium on nutrition tables). Take this into account, slow down your eating, and limit it – share your food with someone.

Make more food at home – you can control the salt content that way.

You'll like raw nuts and seeds just as well when you get used to eating them (doesn't take long).

Remember this: Doing what you've set out to do
benefits you more than anyone else.
And your friends and loved ones will admire you
and like what you've done for yourself.

Binging

Don't. The unfortunate fact of life is that you can put weight back on in 1 day of happy, gluttonous binging that it took you all week to lose and will take you several days to a week to lose again.

If you feel the need to have a lot of pizza during the game Saturday night, eat your healthy breakfast Saturday morning and don't have lunch or have a late breakfast-lunch combination and watch the calories. You may have 1,000 calories or more available for dinner that way. That won't allow for drinking 5 beers and eating a Godzilla-burger or two, but you can allow yourself more flexibility that way. And go walking or doing something physical. That will give you more leeway and up your metabolism to burn off what you eat. Just be sensible. Your body is keeping count even if you forget to.

You'll enjoy your food and drink more if you don't over-indulge – the last bites and drinks are not as good as the first and middle ones when you have a lot.

But . . . if you do overindulge and fall off the wagon, so to speak, don't despair – just pick yourself up and start up again, albeit a few days behind where you were before the over-indulgence.

Snacks

Yes, there's room for snacks. But snack smart. And don't overdo anything.

It's good to keep grapes around at home or watermelon chunks. These are easy to grab, and they're healthy and taste good. Other fruits make good snacks as well.

Raw nuts make good snacks.

So do Clif bars and other energy bars *IF* you can limit yourself to just a *small* bite now and then, 1 or 2 an afternoon, for example. Small bite.

Candy Bars, Chocolate, Big Hamburgers, Pizza, Cheese, Etc.

Most snacks are trouble, the siren song of calories luring you to crash on the rocks like Lorelei to sailors on the Rhine, but you can manage these in extreme moderation. For example, Butterfinger Bites (not bars) – one per week. You really, really like cheese on your sandwich? Put half as much on.

Find a dark chocolate, 70% or more, that you like. Most are bitter. A good one is Trader Joe's Swiss 72%. Dark chocolate has health benefits, and you probably won't eat as much as the milk chocolate ones that are not good for you.

Pizza. Look at it, figure out how much you'd like to eat. Eat one slice less than that. Only occasionally. Or ask them to cut it into 10 slices instead of 8 or 6.

Sure, go out for a big hamburger now and then – just split it with someone.

Same with Chicken Fried Steak.

Fried things? Just pick off some (maybe half) of the fried breading on the outside, and you'll still get the taste of the fried breading along with the shrimp, chicken, or whatever.

Just go easy on these things -- and remember that the sides have calories, too. Give up something for what you like most.

Alcoholic Beverages.

Moderation. Keep track of the calories as you do with food. Quite obviously, this is easy to overdo in more ways than one.

Parties and Celebrations.

These can be alluring sources of calorie temptation. All that food sitting out and an open bar – there's Lorelei again, trying to lure you to crash on the rocks. And with food and drink at hand, these can be as Scylla and Charybdis were for Odysseus in Homer's Odyssey.

Just remember – Moderation -- and -- It All Counts. One way or another, you'll need to give up something. Either eat less before and after or eat and drink less while there. If not, you'll be set back a few days. You can go, drink, eat, and have fun – just be sensible about it.

Chapter 9

Maintenance and Summary

Maintenance.

After you've reached your target weight, set a range you allow yourself to stay within. You probably won't exercise less or walk less, as you've likely incorporated that into your lifestyle. But now you can allow yourself a little more leeway in your eating. A little bit of a large slice, or a very small slice, of pie. 2/3 of that lunch instead of ½.

Just pay attention to your weight. If you find yourself at the top of your own range, back off some on the food and drink (other than water) and add in a little more exercise till you get back to the lower end of your range.

You should be able to stay within a 4 - 5 pound range. For me, that's between 160 and 165 pounds.

Summary.

In general, try to have the majority of your food be fresh fruits, raw nuts, whole grains, pastas, foods that aren't fried, vegetables, foods without a lot of sauce or gravy or cheese, and foods that are healthy, along with eating less and adding exercise you like that's easy to do.

You know when things aren't helping. Your Will Power, your decision making, your inner self will get you through this, and you will be happy you did it and justifiably proud of yourself.

Now get started, and refer to this *Weight Loss – It's Just Nuts* plan frequently. You'll be a happier, slimmer person sooner than you think.

ABOUT THE AUTHOR

Bob Binder is a long time resident of Austin, Texas, and before that, being an Army brat, he lived and grew up in Reno, Texas; Ft. Belvoir, Virginia; West Lafayette, Indiana; Heidelberg, Germany; and Aberdeen, Maryland.

Bob went to college at the University of Texas at Austin for his Bachelor of Business Administration degree and for his Law Degree. He also attended the University of Hawaii one semester.

Having gone through ROTC at the University of Texas, Bob served as an officer at Ft. Gordon, Georgia and in the southern half of Vietnam during the Vietnam War, for which he was awarded a Bronze Star. His subsequent Reserve duty was at Ft. Carson, Colorado over several years and seasons.

Civically, he was elected Student Body President while at the University of Texas and a City Councilmember for Austin, Texas.

Bob became Board Certified in Personal Injury Trial Law and practiced in that capacity representing only plaintiffs for 40 years, and before that he had a varied law practice. He is also a Mediator and has mediated many cases for others to a successful conclusion. His practice has been based in Austin, Texas, except for 9 months in Los Angeles, California (Westwood area) when he lived in Marina del Rey. This practice took Bob throughout Texas, the greater Los Angeles area, and to many states coast to coast besides Texas.

Bob has been in a relationship with Lucile Puett for many years.

Bob has two daughters, Margaux Binder and Paige Binder, who at initial publication live in Seattle, Washington.